THE ULTIMATE 30 DAY PLANT POWERED SMOOTHIE PLAN

Revitalize Your Health and Palate with This 30 Days Delicious Plant-Powered Smoothies, embrace a lifestyle that promotes health, vitality, and environmental consciousness.

ELLIE HOUSTON

TABLE OF CONTENT

INTRODUCTION

Introducing the "30-Day Plant Powered Smoothie Plan" a delectable journey that will rejuvenate your health and tantalize your taste buds. In this comprehensive guide, you'll embark on a month-long adventure of sipping on nutrient-packed, plant-based delights that are not only good for you but also incredibly delicious. Whether you're a seasoned vegan or just beginning to explore the benefits of a plant-powered lifestyle, these easy-to-follow smoothie recipes offer a delightful way to embrace wholesome eating.

Each day, you'll discover a new and exciting smoothie recipe that incorporates a variety of fruits, vegetables, nuts, and superfoods to ensure your palate stays satisfied and your body nourished. From the vibrant green blends to sweet and savory creations, our 30-Day Plant Powered Smoothie Plan is your passport to a healthier, more energized you. Say goodbye to monotony and hello to a month of flavorful exploration as you sip your way to well-being.

30 HEALTHY PLANT-BASED SMOOTHIE PLAN

1 Classic Green Smoothie

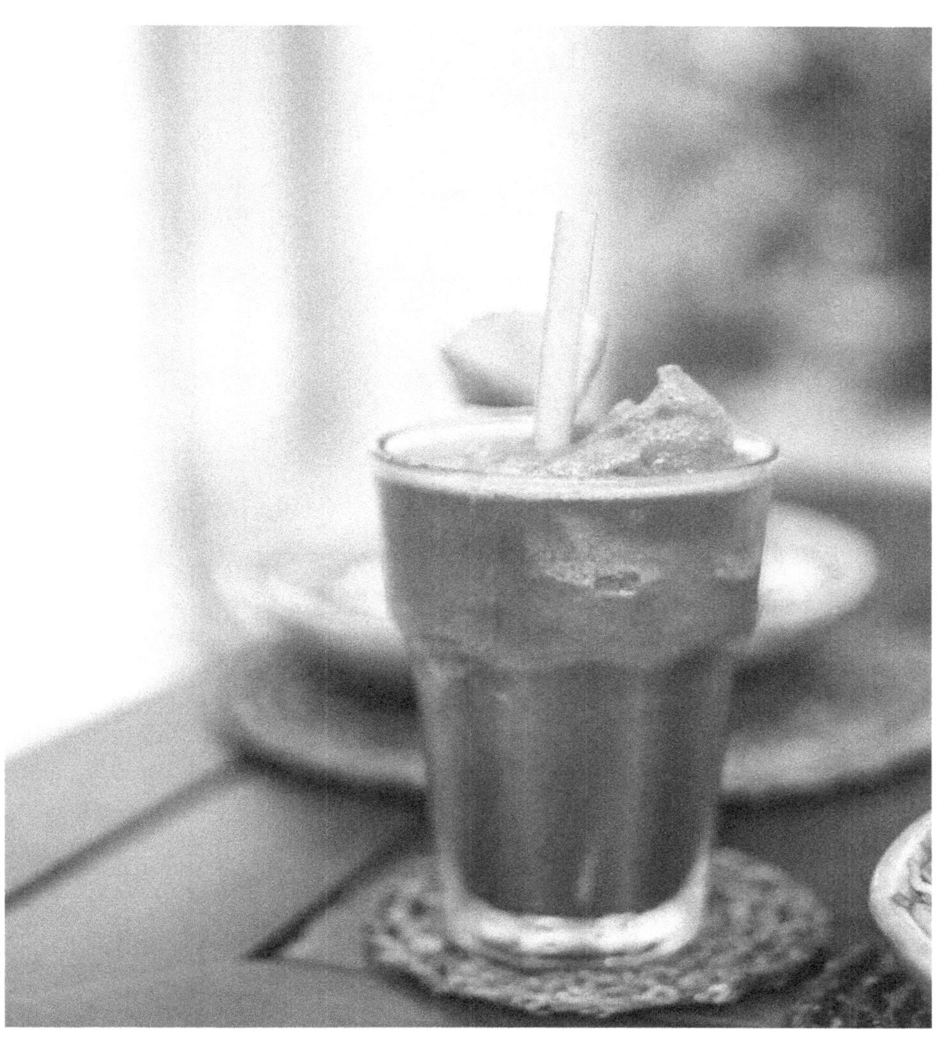

Ingredients:

1 cup of spinach

1 banana

1/2 cup of almond milk

1/2 cup of water

1 tablespoon of chia seeds

Preparation:

Place spinach, banana, almond milk, water, and chia seeds in a blender.

Blend until smooth and creamy. Add more water if needed.

2. *Mango Tango Smoothie*

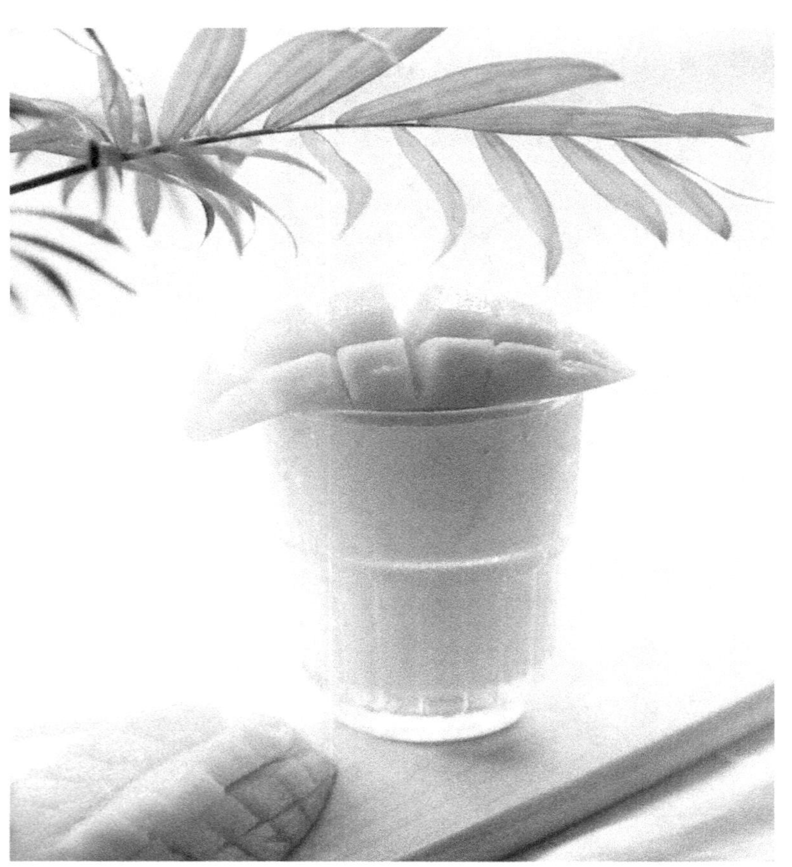

Ingredients:

1 cup of frozen mango chunks

1/2 cup of coconut milk

1/2 cup of orange juice

1 tablespoon of flaxseeds

Preparation:

Combine frozen mango chunks, coconut milk, orange juice, and flaxseeds in a blender.

Blend until smooth and creamy.

3. Berry Bliss Smoothie

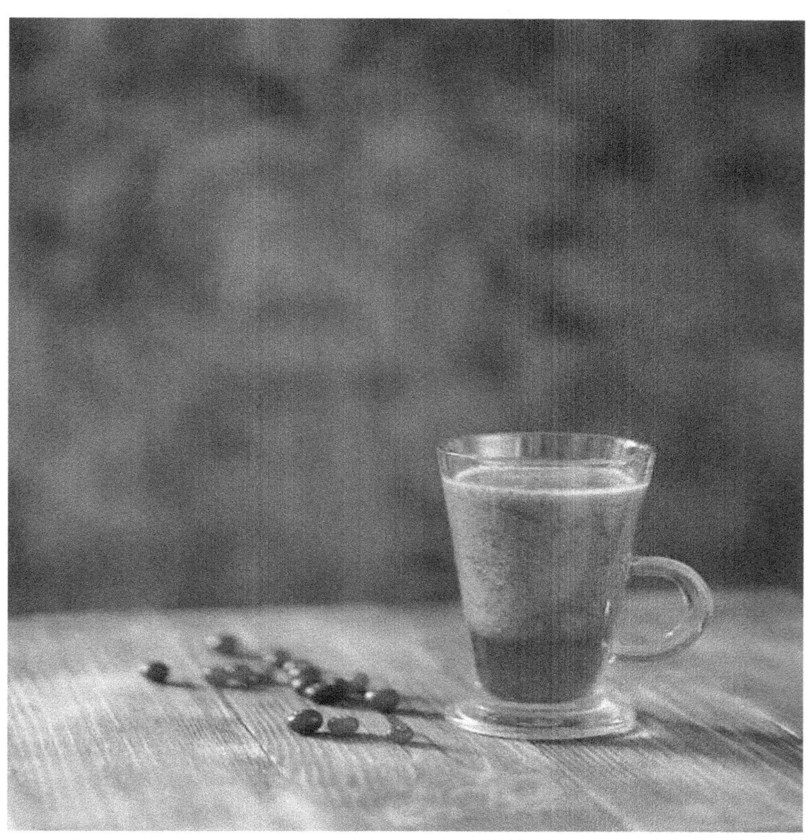

Ingredients:

1 cup of blueberries, raspberries, and strawberries combined

1 banana

1 cup of almond milk

1 tablespoon of maple syrup (optional)

Preparation:

Add mixed berries, banana, almond milk, and maple syrup (if using) to a blender.

Blend until the desired consistency is reached.

4. Creamy Banana Almond Smoothie

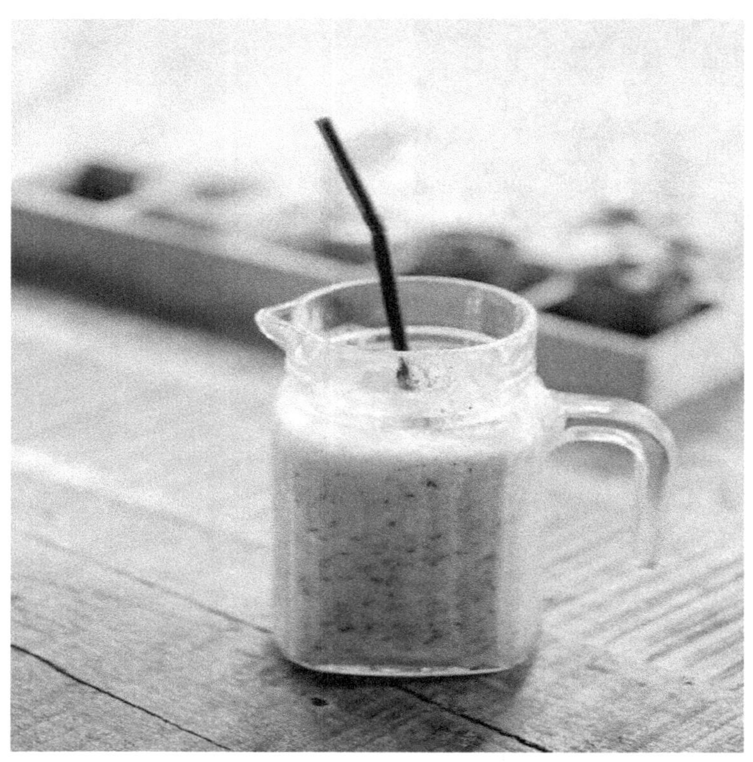

Ingredients:

2 ripe bananas

2 tablespoons of almond butter

1 cup of almond milk

2-3 pitted dates for sweetness (adjust to taste)

A pinch of cinnamon (optional)

Preparation:

Place bananas, almond butter, almond milk, pitted dates, and cinnamon (if using) in a blender.

Blend until smooth and creamy.

5. *Tropical Paradise Smoothie*

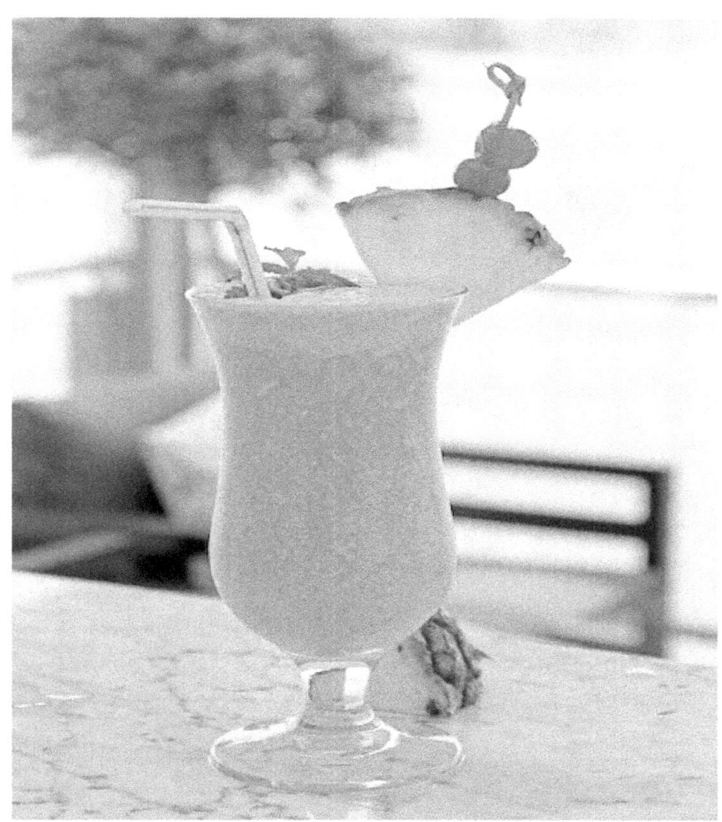

Ingredients:

1 cup of pineapple chunks

1/2 cup of coconut water

1 banana

1 cup of spinach or kale

1 tablespoon of chia seeds

Preparation:

Combine pineapple chunks, coconut water, banana, spinach or kale, and chia seeds in a blender.

Blend until smooth.

6. Peanut Butter & Jelly Smoothie

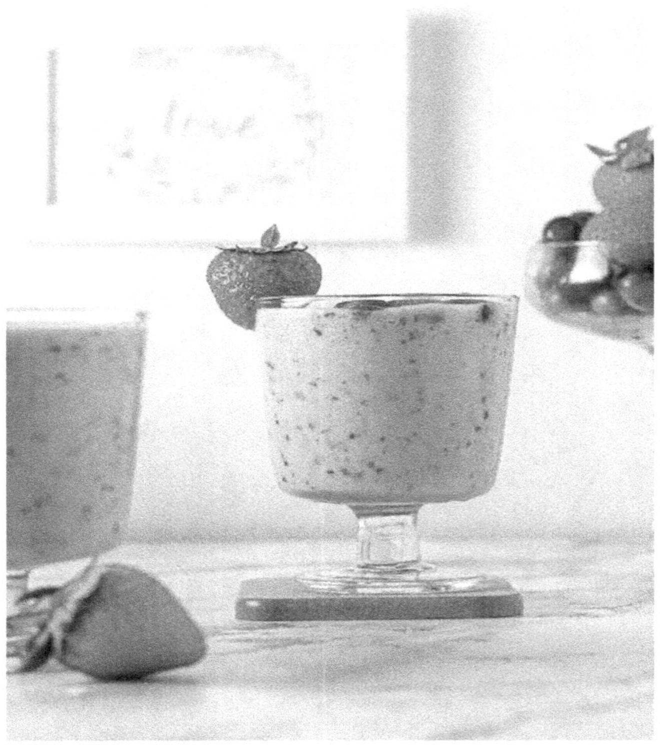

Ingredients:

1 cup of frozen strawberries

1 banana

2 tablespoons of peanut butter

1 cup of almond milk

2 tablespoons of rolled oats

Preparation:

Place frozen strawberries, banana, peanut butter, almond milk, and rolled oats in a blender.

Blend until smooth and creamy.

7. Chocolate Peanut Butter Protein Smoothie

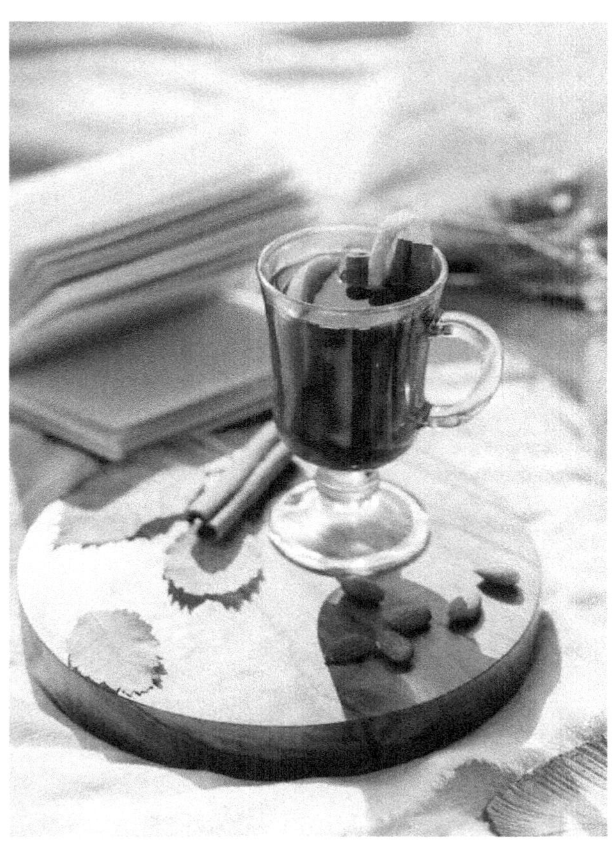

Ingredients:

1 cup of almond milk

1 banana

2 tablespoons of peanut butter

2 tablespoons of unsweetened cocoa powder

1 scoop of plant-based protein powder

Preparation:

Blend almond milk, banana, peanut butter, cocoa powder, and protein powder in a blender until smooth.

8. Blueberry Blast Smoothie

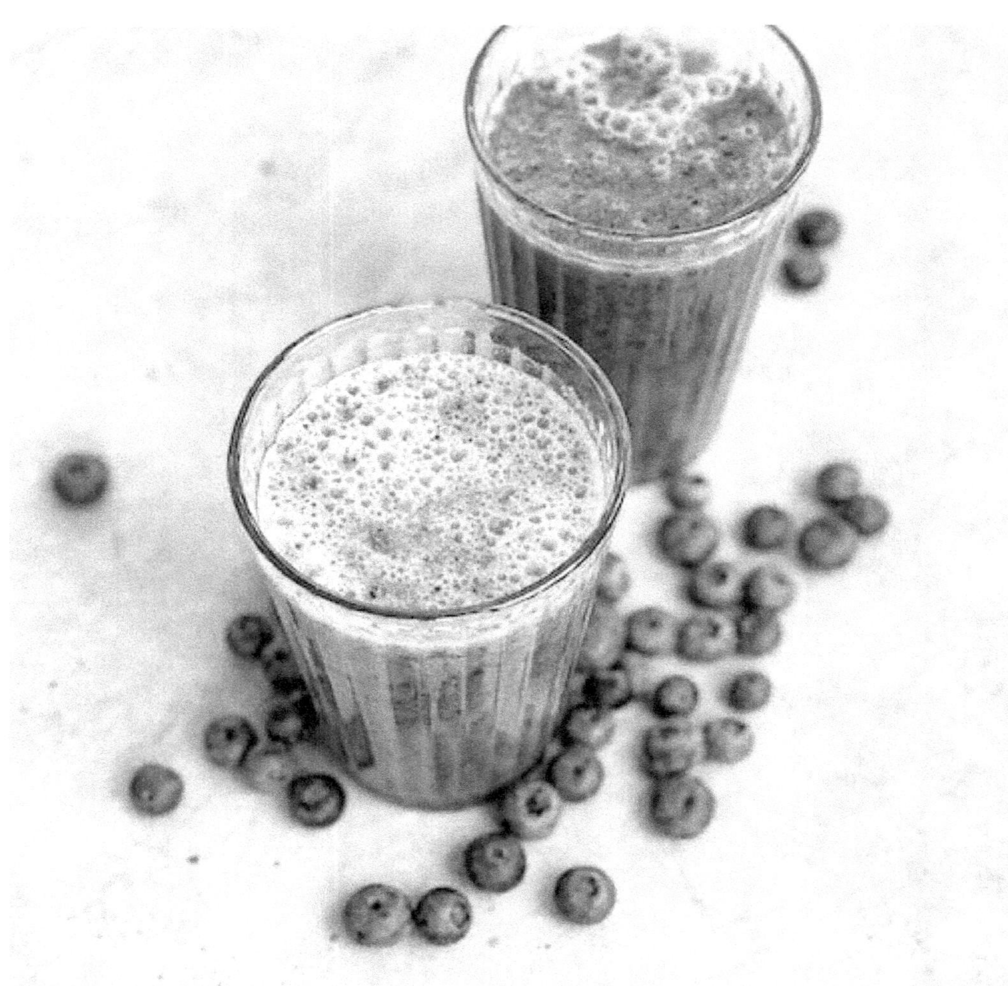

Ingredients:

1 cup of blueberries

1/2 cup of silken tofu

1 cup of almond milk

1 tablespoon of maple syrup

Preparation:

Combine blueberries, silken tofu, almond milk, and maple syrup in a blender.

Blend until smooth and creamy.

9. Avocado Green Smoothie

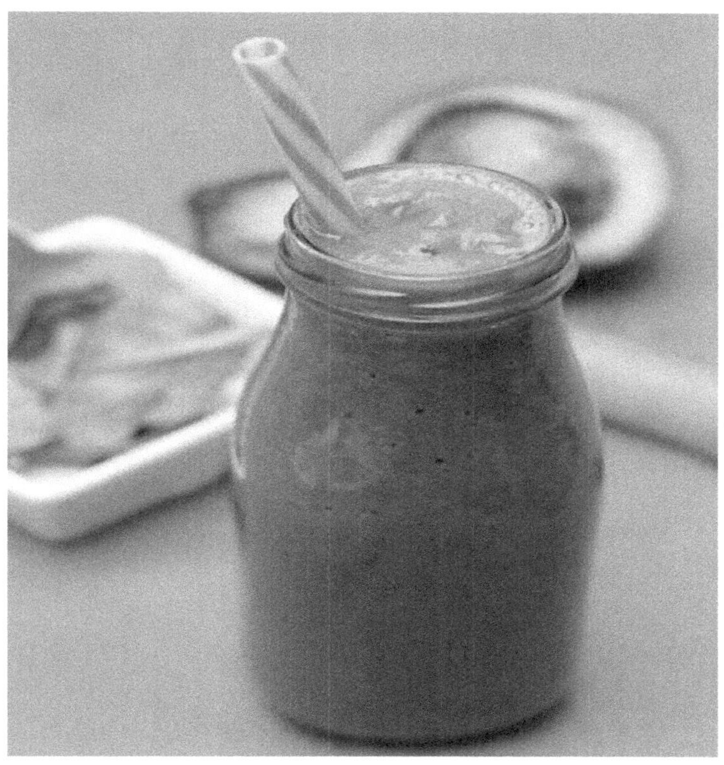

Ingredients:

1/2 avocado

1 cup of spinach

1/2 cup of pineapple chunks

1/2 cup of coconut water

1 tablespoon of chia seeds

Preparation:

Place avocado, spinach, pineapple chunks, coconut water, and chia seeds in a blender.

Blend until smooth and creamy.

10. Raspberry Delight Smoothie

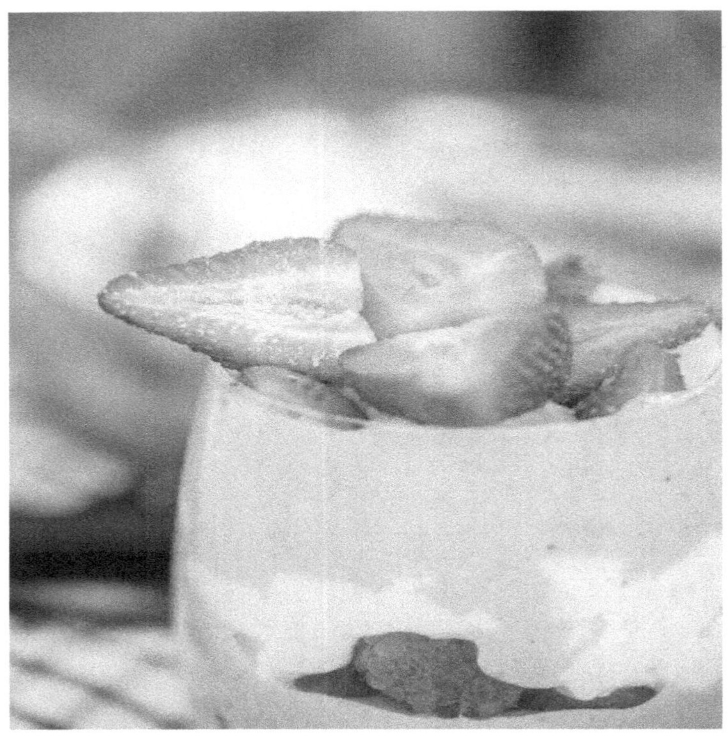

Ingredients:

1 cup of raspberries

1 banana

1 cup of almond milk

1 tablespoon of agave syrup (or any other preferred sweetener)

Preparation:

Add raspberries, banana, almond milk, and agave syrup to a blender.

Blend until you achieve the desired consistency.

11. Chia Cherry Smoothie

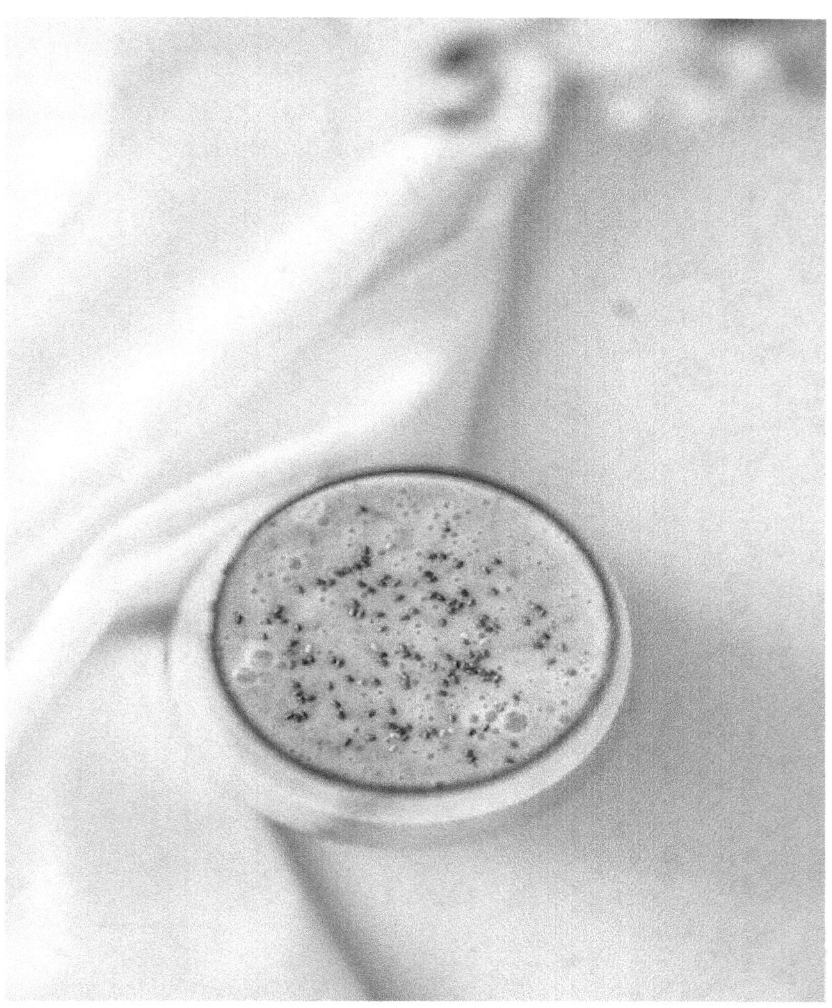

Ingredients:

1 cup of frozen cherries

2 tablespoons of chia seeds

1 cup of almond milk

1 tablespoon of maple syrup

Preparation:

Combine frozen cherries, chia seeds, almond milk, and maple syrup in a blender.

Blend until smooth and thickened by the chia seeds.

12. Spinach and Pineapple Green Smoothie

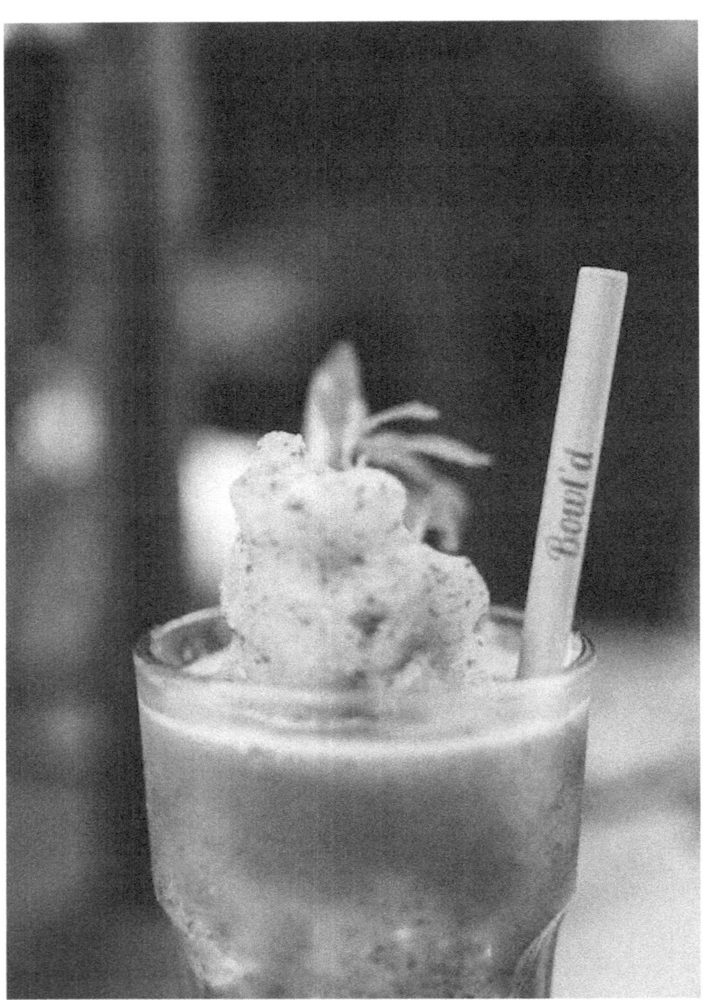

Ingredients:

1 cup of fresh spinach

1 cup of pineapple chunks, either fresh or frozen

1/2 banana

1 cup of coconut water

Preparation:

Place spinach, pineapple chunks, banana, and coconut water in a blender.

Blend until smooth.

13. Oatmeal Cookie Smoothie

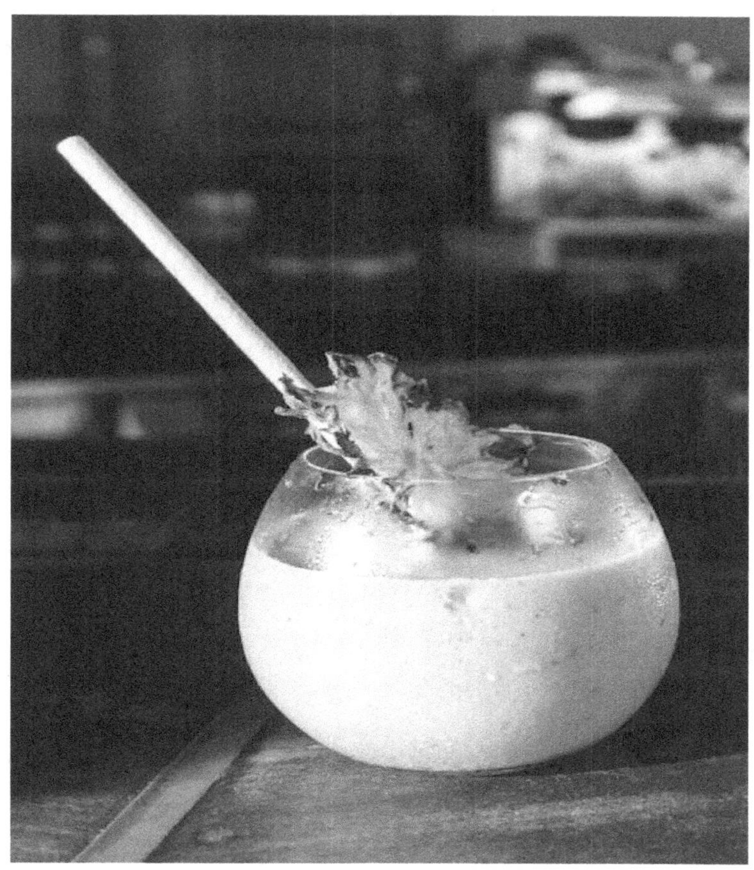

Ingredients:

1/2 cup of rolled oats

1 banana

2 tablespoons of almond butter

1 cup of almond milk

A pinch of cinnamon

Preparation:

Combine rolled oats, banana, almond butter, almond milk, and cinnamon in a blender.

Blend until smooth and creamy.

14. *Almond Joy Smoothie*

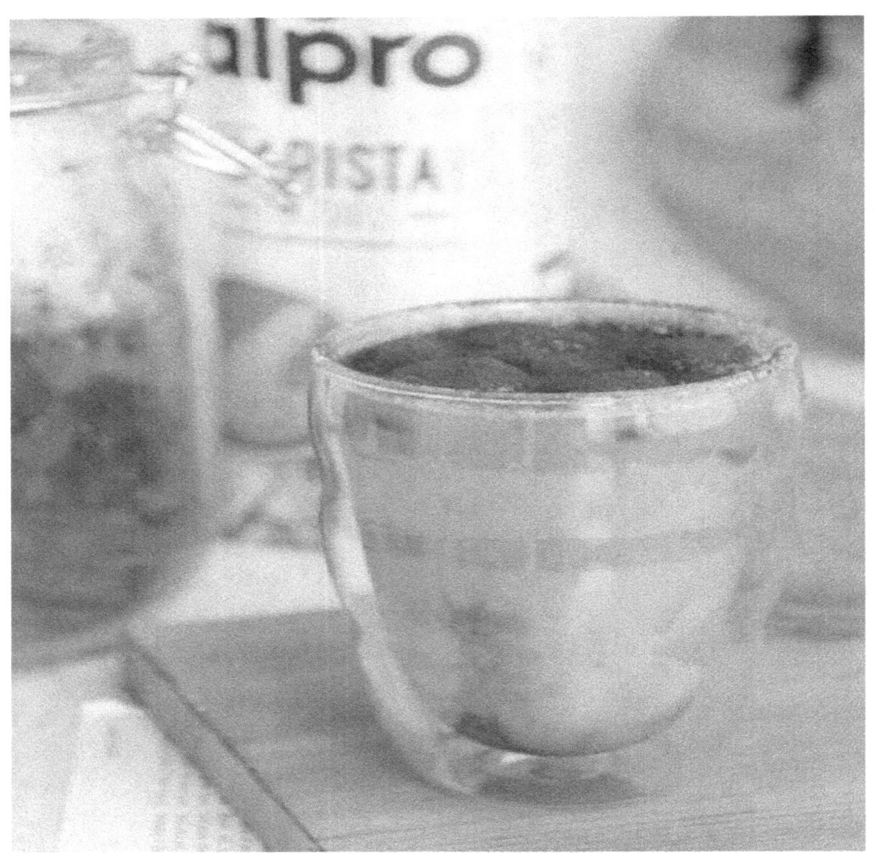

Ingredients:

1 cup of coconut milk

1 banana

2 tablespoons of almond butter

2 tablespoons of cocoa powder

1 tablespoon of shredded coconut

Preparation:

Blend coconut milk, banana, almond butter, cocoa powder, and shredded coconut in a blender until smooth.

15. Creamy Strawberry Banana Smoothie

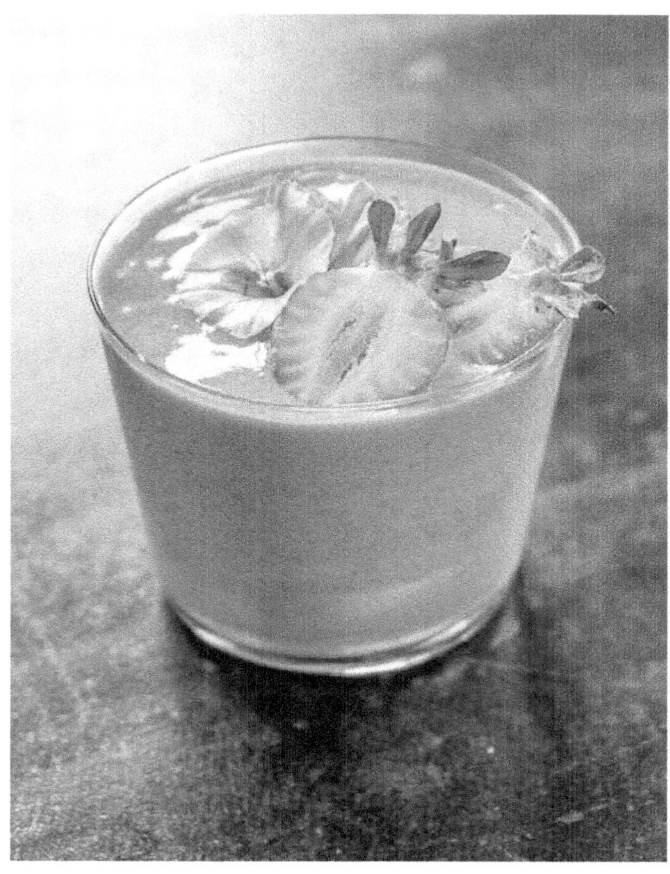

Ingredients:

1 cup of frozen strawberries

1 banana

1 cup of almond milk

1 tablespoon of agave syrup, or any other preferred sweetener

Preparation:

Combine frozen strawberries, banana, almond milk, and agave syrup in a blender.

Blend until smooth and creamy.

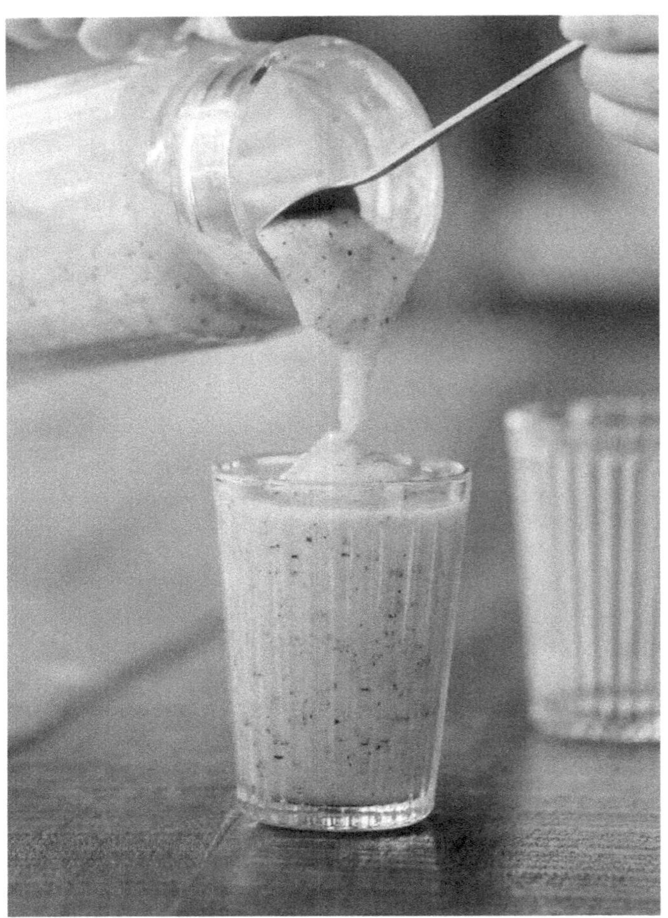

Ingredients:

1 cup of frozen or fresh mango chunks

1 banana

1/2 teaspoon of turmeric

A dash of black pepper (to improve absorption of turmeric)

1 cup of almond milk

Preparation:

Blend mango chunks, banana, turmeric, black pepper, and almond milk in a blender until smooth.

17. *Mint Chocolate Chip Smoothie*

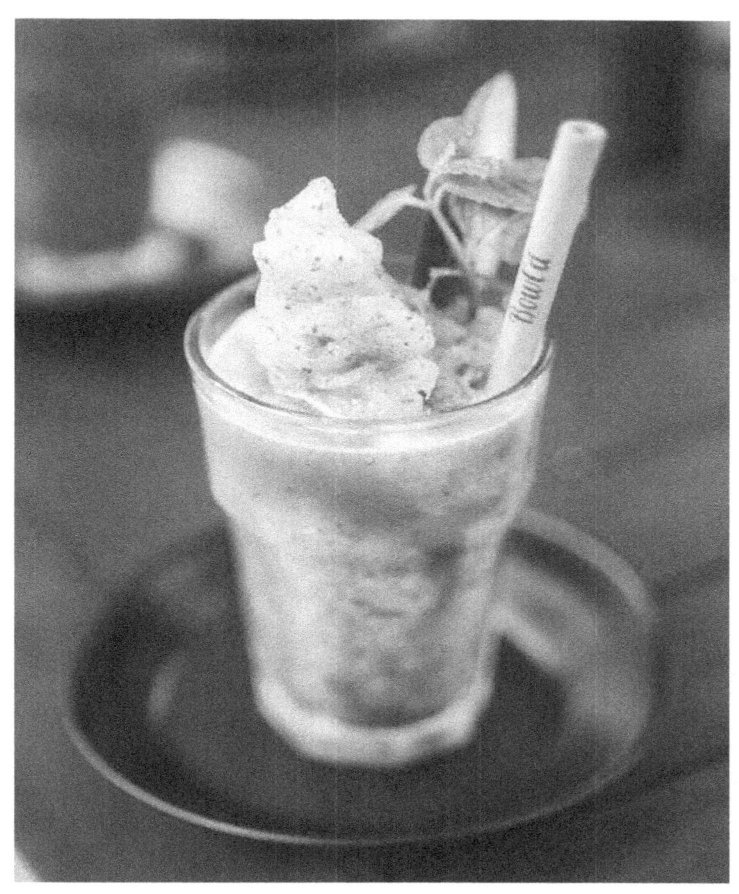

Ingredients:

1 cup of spinach

1/2 avocado

1 tablespoon of cocoa powder

A handful of fresh mint leaves

1 cup of almond milk

1 tablespoon of maple syrup

Preparation:

Place spinach, avocado, cocoa powder, fresh mint leaves, almond milk, and maple syrup in a blender.

Blend until smooth, adjusting the sweetness to your liking.

18. Peanut Butter Cup Smoothie

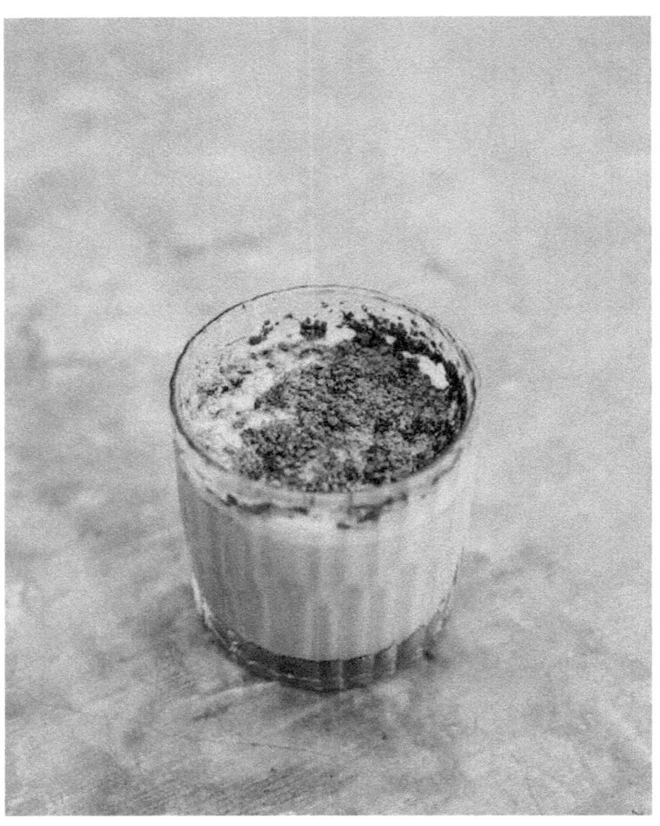

Ingredients:

1 cup of almond milk

1 banana

2 tablespoons of peanut butter

2 tablespoons of cocoa powder

1 tablespoon of agave syrup

Preparation:

Combine almond milk, banana, peanut butter, cocoa powder, and agave syrup in a blender.

Blend until smooth and creamy.

19. Cherry Almond Smoothie

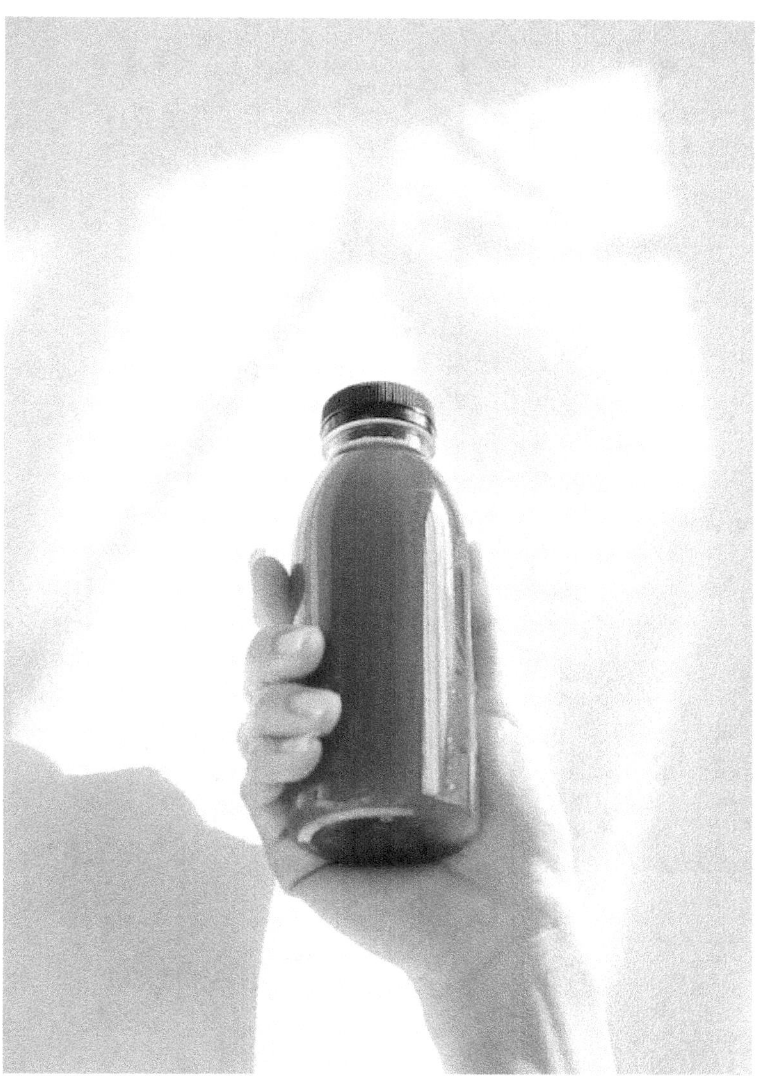

Ingredients:

1 cup of frozen cherries

1/2 cup of almonds

1 cup of almond milk

1 tablespoon of agave syrup

Preparation:

Blend frozen cherries, almonds, almond milk, and agave
syrup in a blender until smooth and creamy.

20. Piña Colada Smoothie

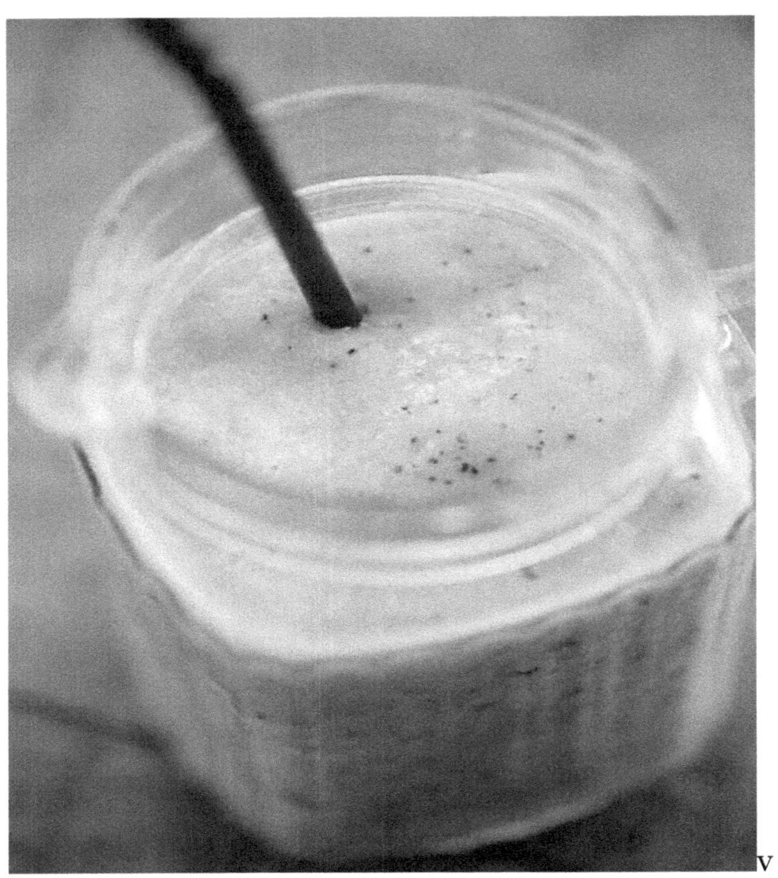

Ingredients:

1 cup of frozen pineapple chunks

1/2 cup of coconut milk

1/2 cup of coconut water

1 banana

A splash of lime juice

Preparation:

Combine frozen pineapple chunks, coconut milk, coconut water, banana, and lime juice in a blender.

Blend until smooth and tropical.

21. Raspberry Chocolate Smoothie

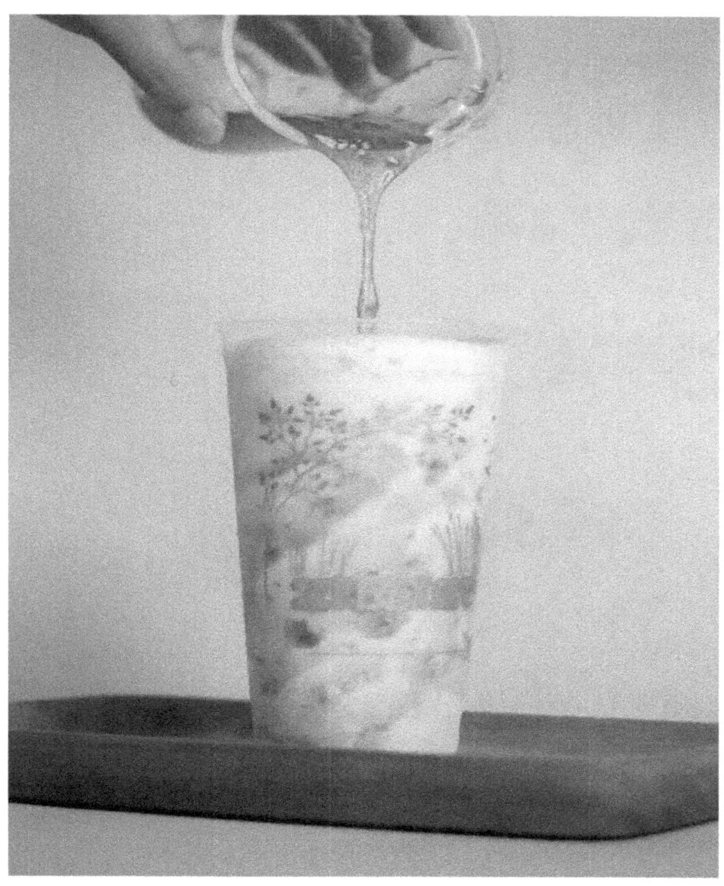

Ingredients:

1 cup of frozen raspberries

1 banana

2 tablespoons of cocoa powder

1 cup of almond milk

1 tablespoon of maple syrup

Preparation:

Blend frozen raspberries, banana, cocoa powder, almond milk, and maple syrup in a blender until smooth and chocolatey.

22. Strawberry Shortcake Smoothie

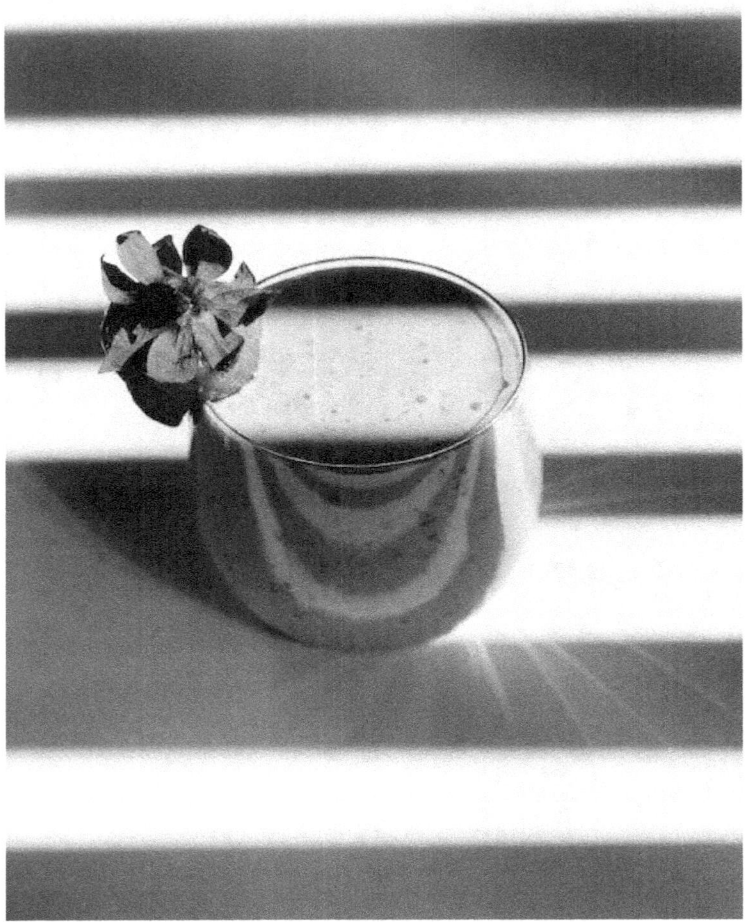

Ingredients:

1 cup of frozen strawberries

1/2 cup of rolled oats

1 cup of almond milk

1 tablespoon of agave syrup, or any other preferred sweetener

Preparation:

Combine frozen strawberries, rolled oats, almond milk, and agave syrup in a blender.

Blend until smooth, with a delightful strawberry shortcake flavor.

23. Matcha Green Tea Smoothie

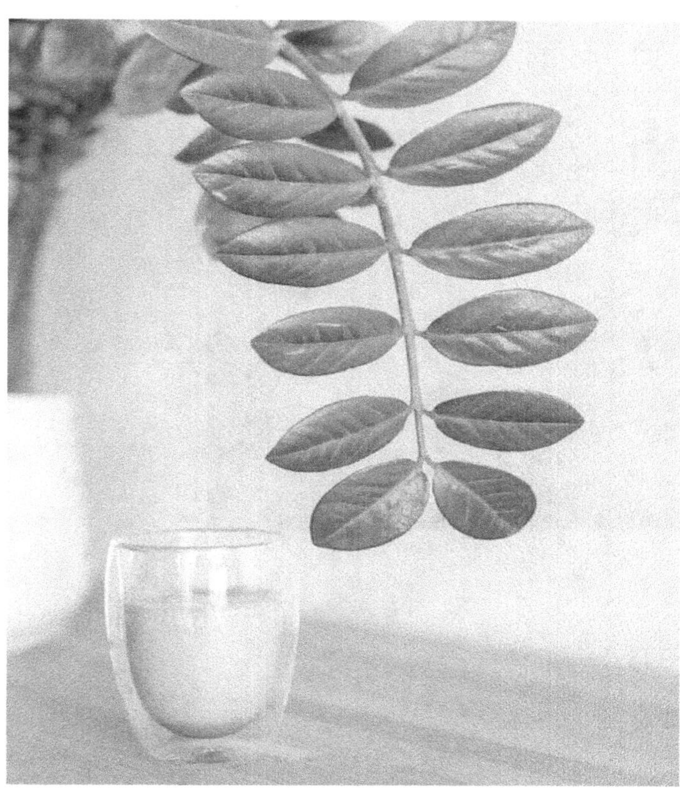

Ingredients:

1 teaspoon of matcha powder

1 banana

1 cup of almond milk

1 tablespoon of agave syrup, or any other preferred sweetener

Preparation:

Blend matcha powder, banana, almond milk, and agave syrup in a blender until smooth and green.

24. Pumpkin Pie Smoothie

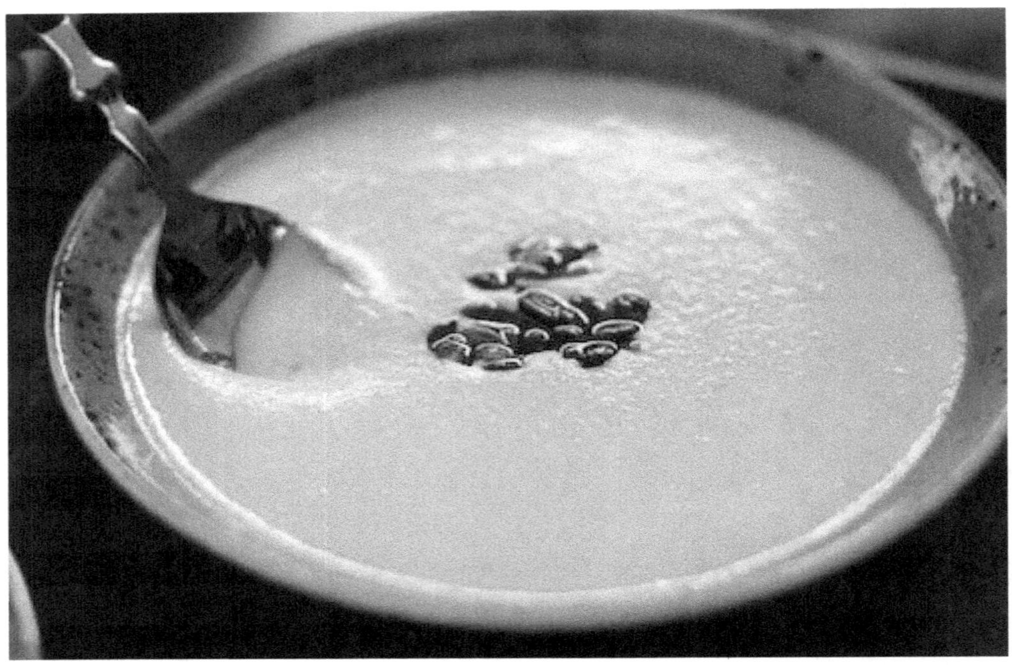

Ingredients:

1/2 cup of canned pumpkin puree

1 banana

1/2 teaspoon of pumpkin pie spice

1 cup of almond milk

1 tablespoon of maple syrup

Preparation:

Combine pumpkin puree, banana, pumpkin pie spice, almond milk, and maple syrup in a blender.

Blend until smooth, reminiscent of a pumpkin pie.

25. Kiwi Kale Smoothie

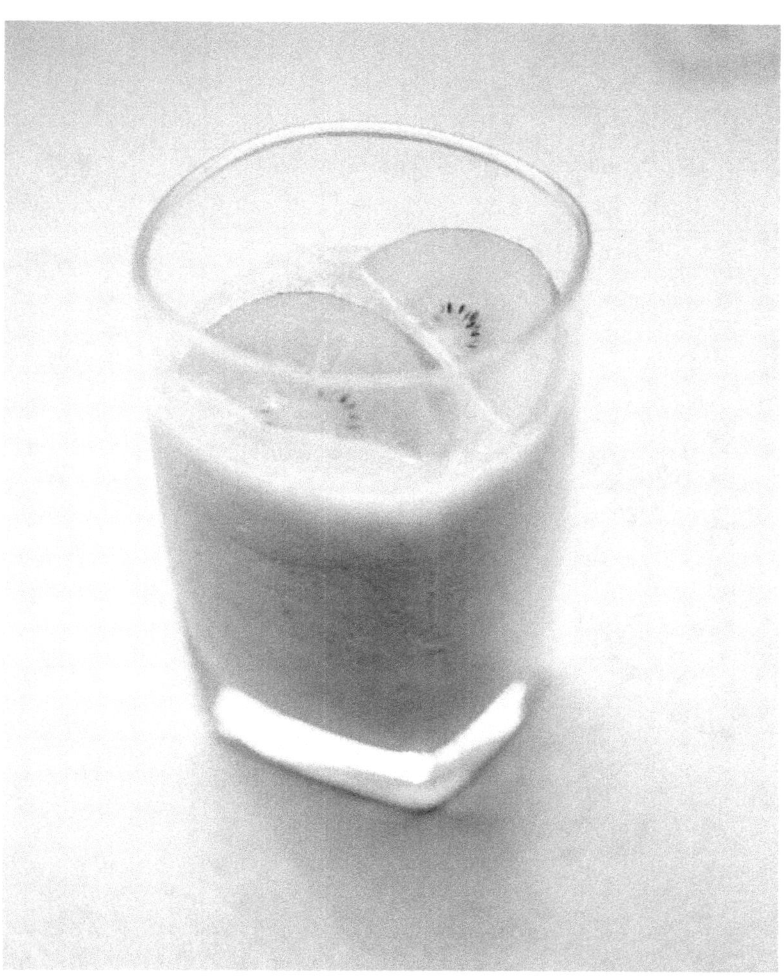

Ingredients:

2 kiwis, peeled and sliced

1 cup of kale leaves (stems removed)

1 banana

1 cup of coconut water

Preparation:

Place kiwi, kale leaves, banana, and coconut water in a blender.

Blend until smooth, yielding a vibrant green smoothie.

26. Blueberry Muffin Smoothie

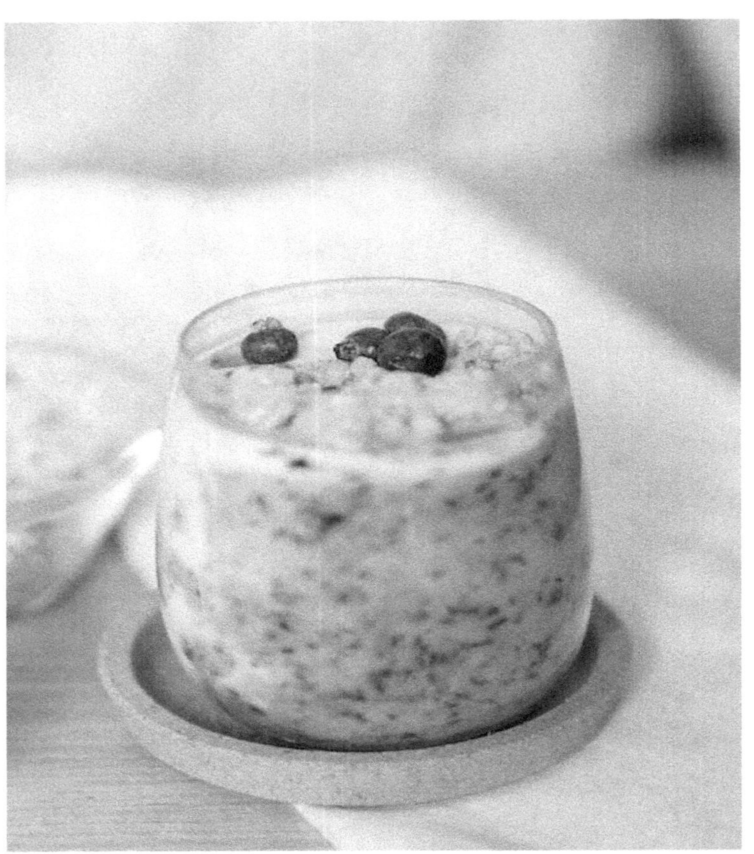

Ingredients:

1 cup of frozen blueberries

1/2 cup of rolled oats

1 cup of almond milk

A pinch of cinnamon

One tablespoon of agave syrup, or any other preferred sweetener

Preparation:

Blend frozen blueberries, rolled oats, almond milk, agave syrup, and a pinch of cinnamon in a blender until smooth and reminiscent of a blueberry muffin.

27. Banana Chocolate Chip Smoothie

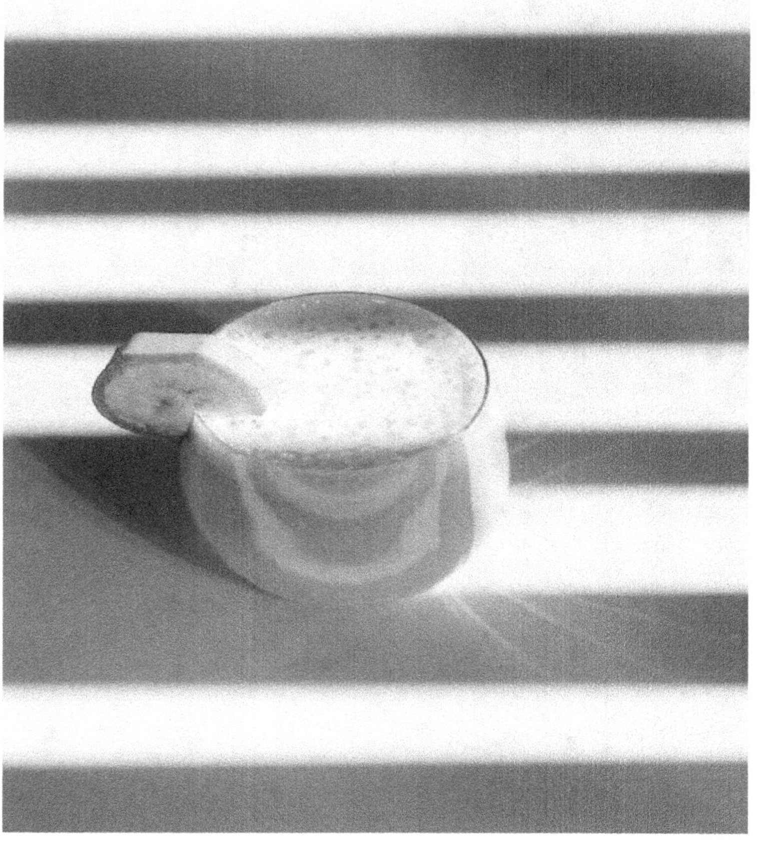

Ingredients:

2 bananas

2 tablespoons of cocoa nibs or vegan chocolate chips

1 cup of almond milk

1 tablespoon of agave syrup, or any other preferred sweetener

Preparation:

Combine bananas, cocoa nibs or chocolate chips, almond milk, and agave syrup in a blender.

Blend until smooth, creating a banana-chocolate delight.

28. Orange Creamsicle Smoothie

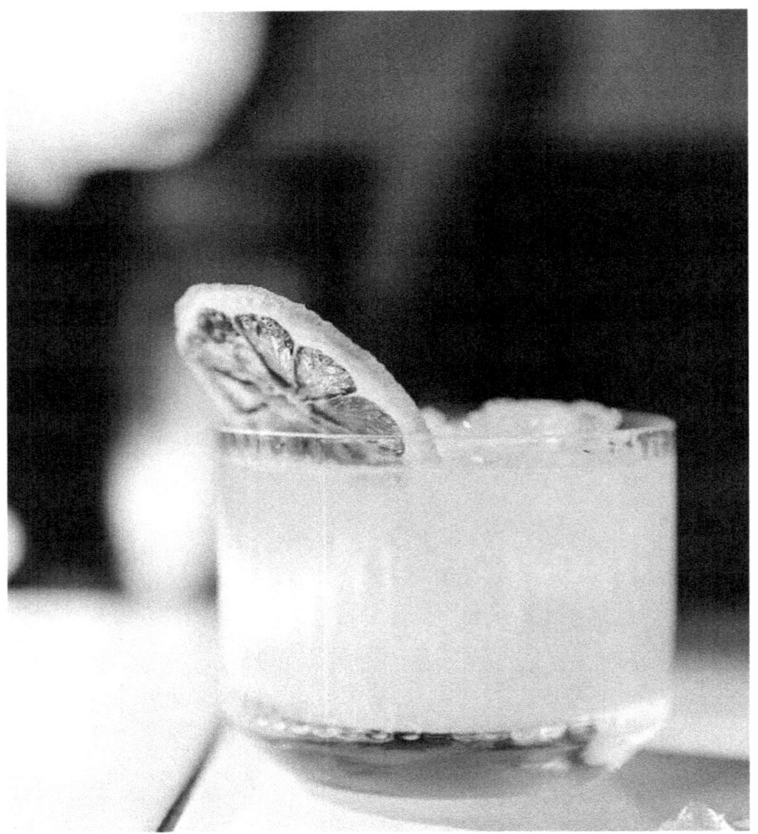

Ingredients:

2 oranges, peeled and segmented

1 banana

1/2 cup of coconut milk

1/2 cup of almond milk

1 tablespoon of agave syrup

Preparation:

Place orange segments, banana, coconut milk, almond milk, and agave syrup in a blender.

Blend until smooth and reminiscent of an orange creamsicle.

29. Cucumber Lime Cooler Smoothie

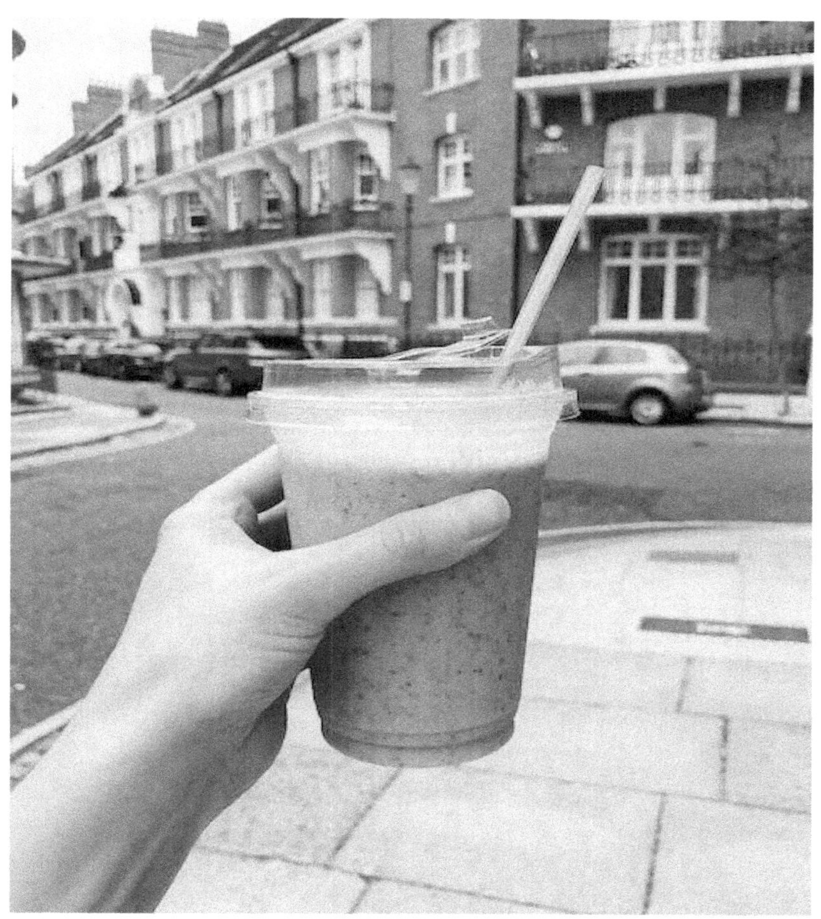

Ingredients:

1 cucumber, peeled and sliced

Juice of 2 limes

1 banana

1 cup of coconut water

Fresh mint leaves (for garnish)

Preparation:

Combine cucumber slices, lime juice, banana, and coconut water in a blender.

Blend until smooth, and garnish with fresh mint leaves.

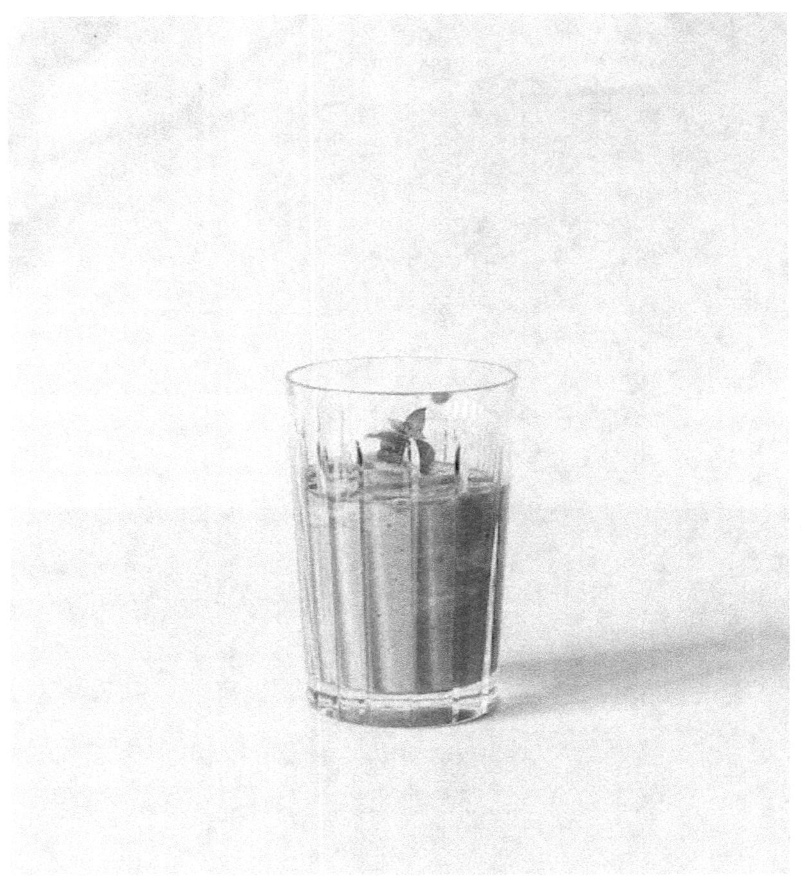

Ingredients:

2 cups of fresh watermelon chunks

1/2 cup of fresh basil leaves

Juice of 1 lime

1 tablespoon of agave syrup

Ice cubes

Preparation:

Place watermelon chunks, basil leaves, lime juice, agave syrup, and ice cubes in a blender.

Blend until smooth, creating a refreshing and unique watermelon basil smoothie.

CONCLUSION

As you reach the culmination of your 30-Day Plant Based Smoothie Plan, it's time to reflect on the remarkable journey you've undertaken. You've not only indulged in a symphony of tantalizing flavors but also embraced a lifestyle that promotes health, vitality, and environmental consciousness.

Throughout this month, you've witnessed the transformative power of whole, plant-based foods, and the impact they can have on your well-being. These smoothies have nourished your body with essential vitamins, minerals, and antioxidants, leaving you feeling more energetic and rejuvenated.

The beauty of this plan is that it's not limited to just 30 days; it's a gateway to a lifelong commitment to better health and ethical choices. You've explored a rainbow of ingredients, and you've learned that healthy eating can be an exciting and delicious adventure.

As you conclude this journey, remember that the vibrant flavors and benefits of these smoothies can continue to be a part of your daily life. Cheers to a healthier, kinder, and more vibrant you!